Home Remedies

For Cancer

Home Remedies
For Cancer

By Monica Sidoine,
S.N.H.S. Dip. Herbalism

DISCLAIMER

This book is to serve as an informational guide for use in the home. The remedies and procedures contained in this book are meant to supplement and are not intended to be a substitute for professional medical care. Please seek a qualified medical practitioner for all ailments. The author nor distributors takes no responsibility for customers choosing to treat themselves. Your use of this information is at your own risk.

ISBN - 13: 978-1533557650
ISBN - 10: 1533557659

Proof Read by Jasmine Ned Anunda

Published By Create Space Publishing
United States of America

ACKNOWLEDGMENTS

I would like to thank all those who have contributed in one way or another to the completion of HOME REMEDIES FOR CANCER.

I thank God for giving me the vision, wisdom and good health to write this book. For all he has done and will continue to do in my life.

For the many prayer warriors who interceded on behalf of this project and also their moral support.

I thank my daughter Jasmine Ned Anunda for proof reading.

Thank you all.

Monica Sidoine.

PREFACE

The procedures in this Book was designed to be as simple as possible so that anyone will be able to follow them. Most of the items used are local things which you would either have at home, in your kitchen garden or can be easily purchased from the local market or health store for a very low cost.

TABLE OF CONTENTS

Acknowledgements 5

Preface...7

Cancer 10

    Breast 16

    Colon 20

    Prostate 22

    Skin 25

CANCER

Cancer is a malignant tumor or growth caused when cells multiply uncontrollably destroying healthy tissue.

NATURAL REMEDIES

- Boil 1oz of red clover seeds in 1 liter of water for 30 minutes. Drink 5 cups daily.

- Steep 5 neem leaves to 2 cups of boiling water for 30 minutes.
  Drink 1 cup twice daily.

- Simmer 4 teaspoons of turmeric powder in 5 cups of boiling water for 5 minutes.
  Drink 1 cup 4 times daily before meals and at bedtime.

- Take ½ cup noni juice and lots of carrot juice daily.

- Peel and chop 2lb of cantaloupe, squeeze 2lb of oranges.
  Blend the cantaloupe and orange juice together. Serve cold.
  Drink 1 glass ½ hour before each meal.

- Green smoothie: 1 cup parsley, ½ cup lemon juice, ¾ cup pineapple juice, 3 stalks celery, 1 carrot, ¼ cup sunflower seeds. Blend all the ingredients and add 1 tablespoon ground flaxseed.

- Hemoglobin booster: 1 beet or 1 carrot, I cup spinach, 1 tablespoon annatto seed, 1 cup water. Blend all the ingredients together.

- Aloe juice: 1 aloe leaf with the skin, remove the prickles. Blend it along with 4 cups of water.
  Take ½ cup with breakfast and lunch.

- Grape juice: 20oz grape juice, 20 okras. Blend all the ingredients together.
  Take ½ cup with breakfast and lunch.

- Garlic juice: 3 cloves of garlic, ½ of a lemon or ½ cup tomato juice or celery juice. Blend the ingredients together.
  Take ½ cup with each meal.

- Green drink: Juice or blend a combination of green vegetables.

- Soybean drink: ½ cup soya milk, put 1 tablespoon ground flaxseed or flaxseed oil on top of the milk.
  Take ½ cup with breakfast and lunch.

- Chia gel: 7 tablespoons chia seeds, 3 ½ cups water. Combine and stir till it starts to get thick. Leave it for 24 hours before serving.
  Take 3 tablespoons with each meal.

- Drink 4 cups of carrot juice and 2 cups of green drink daily.

- Juice wheat grass and drink daily.

- Drink water daily.
  A normal adult under 50 years: 8-10 glasses, over 50 years: 10-12 glasses.

- Eat soursop fruit.

- Eat pineapple to break the membranes of the cancer cells.

- Eat three cloves of raw garlic three times daily.

- Eat three steamed garlic cloves with ¼ lemon squeezed over it with each meal or 4 garlic capsules 4 times daily.

- **For serious Cancer stages:**
  I whole bulb of steamed or lightly baked garlic with each meal.

- Eat lots of raw onions, parsley and cilantro.

- Eat lots of raw food.

- For the first three months of the treatment period 50-80% of the meal should be eaten raw.

- Go on an all raw diet for one month using foods that are bright yellow or dark green.

- Use only whole grains.

- Use aloe and lemons.

- Have a diet high in seeds, nuts, vegetables and fruits, especially deep yellow fruits and vegetables. The cabbage family – Brussels sprouts, broccoli, radish, cabbage, collards, mustard greens, kale, turnip, cauliflower. Beets, carrots, asparagus, dark greens watercress, sunflower seeds, almonds, peanuts, avocado, olives, coconut, grapes, blueberries, cherries, muscadines, cranberries.

- Apply a red clover seed fomentation on the cancerous growths.

HERBAL TEA FOMENTATION:

1. Boil 1oz of red clover seeds in 1 liter of water for 30 minutes.
2. Dip a towel folded in 2 or 3 layers the size of the body area you want to cover in the solution.
3. Wring out the excess liquid. Apply it to the affected area of the body.
4. Place a thick towel over the fomentation to help retain the heat longer.
5. Keep the tea hot and change the cloths every 3 minutes. Do 5 rounds.
6. End with a cold towel rub to the area.

- Apply a poultice of red clover seeds to the cancerous growths.
  Boil some seeds, mash them and add a little warm water to make a paste.

- Follow a two meal plan daily if you can.

- Have a heavy breakfast and lunch.

- If you are having supper it should be very light such as bread, whole grains or fruit.

- Fast 1-3 meals weekly. On the fasting day for breakfast and lunch you can have 2 celery stalks, pineapple or cantaloupe, 1 tablespoon ground flaxseed, 2 tablespoon chia gel. For supper 1 grapefruit, 1 apple, 1 tablespoon chia gel.

Health tips

- Eat slowly, and chew well.

- Do not overeat.

- Have at least five hours between the end of one meal and the beginning of the next meal.

- Avoid rancid fats and foods, burned foods.

- Avoid irritants such as spicy foods, pepper, vinegar, etc.

- Avoid fermented foods.

- No red meat, chicken, fish.

- No eggs, milk, cheese, animal products - sodium caseinate, gelatin, mono & di-glycerides.

- No sugar, sweets, chocolate, fats, limit sweets.

- No white rice, white bread, white flour products.

- No MSG-monosodium glutamate, baking soda-sodium bicarbonate.

- No coffee, soft drinks, ice cream.

- No tobacco, caffeine, nicotine, alcohol.

- No refined foods.

- No smoked or cured foods.

- No oils, margarine, shortening, greases, fried foods.

- Do not eat fruits and vegetables at the same meal.

- Avoid canned food, especially canned tomatoes.

- Avoid farmed salmon.

- Avoid Hydrogenated Oil.

- Avoid Potato Chips.

- Genetically Modified Foods (GMOs)

BREAST CANCER

Some of the symptoms are:-
Lumps in the breast that are firm and don't go away, pain in the breast or chest area, itching, soreness and redness of the nipple, sensitive nipples, nipple discharge, changes in breast appearance, pain in upper back, neck and shoulder.

Some risk factors are:-
Overweight, very large breasts, large waist circumference, early onset of menstrual periods, late menopause, became obese after menopause, giving birth to children at a late age, not bearing children, children who were born overweight, the use of contraceptives, persons having abortions under the age of 18 or over the age of 30 or after 8 weeks gestation, obesity, a family history of breast cancer, history of alcoholism and eating a high fat diet, taller women, nipple secretions, low thyroid activity, a sedentary lifestyle, excessive drinking, exposure to radiation, hormone replacement therapy during menopause, ionizing radiation.

Women who eat eggs daily have a 3.8 times higher breast cancer risk than those who eat eggs less than once a week. Have a 3 times higher fatal ovarian cancer rate than those who eat eggs less than once a week.

NATURAL REMEDIES

- Boil 1oz of red clover seed in 1 liter of water for 20 minutes. Drink 1 cup three times daily.

- Boil 1oz of burdock in 1 liter of water for 20 minutes. Drink 1 cup three times daily.

- Steep 1oz of milk thistle in 1 liter of boiling water for 20 minutes. Drink 1 cup three times daily.

Health Tips

- Make sure that your diet consists of nuts, seeds, broccoli, vegetables and fruits especially oranges and grapefruits, grapes, watermelon, peanuts, tomatoes, soybeans and yellow vegetables.

- Have flaxseed.

- Get extra fiber in your diet.

- Drink water daily. A normal adult under 50 years: 8-10 glasses, over 50 years: 10-12 glasses.

- Keep the arms and the legs warm if the environment is cold.

- Have sunlight.

- Do outdoor walking at least 4 times weekly.

- Perform breast self-exams once every two months.

- Avoid dairy products.

- Avoid meat.

- Avoid alcohol.

- Avoid caffeine or nicotine.

- Do not overeat.

- Achieve your ideal weight.

- Wash and rinse the breast gently.

- Exercise daily for at least 30 minutes.

- Get at least 8 hours of sleep.

- Do not avoid breastfeeding your babies.

- Avoid sugar, honey, and molasses.

- Avoid vinegar.

- Avoid hot spices.

- Do not consume too much peanut.

- Do not consume too much soy products.

- Avoid permanent dark hair dyes.

- Avoid hormone treatments.

- Limit postmenopausal hormone therapy.

- Avoid contraceptives

- Avoid exposure to radiation.

- Avoid exposure to chemicals that can cause cancer.

- Avoid supplements containing iron.

- Avoid wearing a bra for more than 12 hours a day.

- Avoid bras which have the stiffening wires in them.

COLON CANCER

The development of malignant cells in the large intestine lining.

Some of the symptoms are:-
Passing out blood in the stool.
Constipation, rectal bleeding.
Paleness, anemia.
Gas pains, abdominal pains and tenderness.
Changes in bowel habits, bloating.
Weight loss, fatigue.

Some risk factors are:-
Personal or family history of cancer.
Polyps of the colon or rectum.
Inflammatory bowel disease.

Other factors are:-
Chlorinated water, hot spices, pepper, cayenne, high fat diet, especially animal fats, alcoholic beverages, smoking, the intake of high amounts of dietary iron, early onset of menstrual periods, family history of breast or colon cancer, overeating, obesity, lack of exercise.

Women eating the highest amounts of red meats, sweets, french fries and refined grains had 1.5 times the risk of colon cancer of women who ate more fruits, vegetables, fish and whole grains.

Health Tips

- Deseed and chop 2 apples and two avocados. Blend them along with 1 cup of coconut milk and 2 tablespoons of honey until very smooth.
Serve cold.

- Eat 4 ½ lbs. of apples a day for 3 to 5 consecutive days. Water may be drunk. The apples may be eaten raw, as applesauce, baked or cooked but without additional sweeteners.
This treatment may be repeated several times a year.

- Eat 3 cloves of raw garlic with each meal daily.

- Eat ¼ cup of cooked soybeans daily.

- Eat a high fiber diet.

- Same treatment as for Cancer.

- Avoid barbequed foods.

- Avoid fried foods.

- Avoid iron and Vitamin D supplements.

PROSTATE CANCER

Some of the symptoms are:-
Urinating frequently.
Pain or burning sensation when urinating.
Having trouble to urinate.
A decrease in the amount of urine flow.
Blood in the urine.
Lower back or pelvic pain.

Some of the causes are:-
The use of dairy products.
The use of meat and a high fat diet.
An increased heart rate due to the lack of exercise.
An over active sex life.
The use of alcohol, smoking.
The use of drug diuretics.
Occupational exposure to asbestos, steel, iron, nickel, lead, fertilizer, bitumen pitch, lacquers and dyes.
Family history of prostate cancer.
Some diseases such as heart disease, kidney stones, hypertension, chronic bronchitis, rheumatic disease, tuberculosis, diabetes.

NATURAL REMEDIES

- Boil 1oz of red clover seed in 1 liter of water for 20 minutes. Drink 1 cup three times daily.

- Boil 1oz of black cohosh in 1 liter of water for 20 minutes. Drink 1 cup three times daily.

- Steep 1oz of angelica in 1 liter of boiling water for 20 minutes.
  Drink 1 cup three times daily.

- Boil 1oz of Echinacea in 1 liter of water for 20 minutes. Drink 1 cup three times daily.

- Boil 1oz of goldenseal in 1 liter of water for 20 minutes. Drink 1 cup three times daily.

- Steep 1oz of saw palmetto in 1 liter of boiling water for 20 minutes.
  Drink 1 cup three times daily.

- Boil 1oz of burdock in 1 liter of water for 20 minutes. Drink 1 cup three times daily.

- Boil 1oz of turmeric in 1 liter of water for 20 minutes. Drink 1 cup three times daily.

- Eat lycopene rich foods:–
  Watermelon, strawberries, pink grapefruit, red guava, apricot, tomatoes.

- Eat selenium rich foods: –
  Oatmeal, sunflower seeds, barley.

- Eat legumes: –
  Garbanzo beans, beans, soybeans, lentils, peas, lima beans.

- Eat Vitamin E rich foods: –
  Wheat germ, beans, avocado, seeds, almonds, olives.

- Eat ½ cup of soybeans daily.

- Eat the pectin from citrus fruits.

- Drink fresh fruit and vegetable juices daily.
  Especially carrot, beet, and cabbage juices.

Health Tips

- Take at least 20 minutes of sunlight early in the morning.

- Exercise daily for at least 30 minutes.

SKIN CANCER

Skin cancer is categorized as either Melanoma or Non-Melanoma. The major risk factor is over exposure to the sunlight and it appears on body surfaces which are most frequently exposed.

Some of the signs are:-
Changes in the colour or size of a mole.
Change in a wart.
Change in a growth or darkly pigmented spot.
Some reddish spots on the chest, shoulder, arm or leg.
Change in sensation.
Itchiness, tenderness, or pain.
Bleeding, oozing or scaliness.
Spread of pigmentation beyond its borders.
An open sore that bleeds, crusts over and it will not heal properly.

NATURAL REMEDIES

- Boil 1oz of red clover seeds in 1 liter of water for 20 minutes. Drink 1 cup three times daily.

- Boil 1oz of burdock root in 1 liter of water for 20 minutes. Drink 1 cup three times daily.

- Steep 1oz of chaparral in 1 liter of boiling water for 20 minutes.
  Drink 1 cup three times daily.

- Drink ½ cup blended aloe 3 times daily for months.

- Go on an all raw food diet for one month.

- Take 2 tablespoons of flaxseed oil daily.

- Apply the milky sap from the soursop on the skin cancer or warts on the skin of the soles, palms or hairy skin surfaces.
  Do three treatments of it. One every other day.

- Cut a thin slice of garlic and apply it with a tape over the area. If you put one on in the morning remove it in the evening and put a fresh one for the night. Wash the area after every change.
  Do it for four days. After that allow the area to heal, if there are any remains repeat the treatment in about three weeks' time.

- Apply a solution of myrrh or goldenseal to the areas which are affected.

Health Tips

- Get enough rest.

- Get your sunlight before 10.00 am. and after 4.00 pm.

- Use an SPF15 sunscreen.

- When you are out in the sun wear protective clothing.

- Wear light coloured clothing.

- Eat an adequate amount of essential fatty acids.

- Same treatment as for Cancer.

Other Book Titles by the Same Author

Can be viewed at this link:
http://www.amazon.com/author/monicasidoine

Home Remedies For Stress, Depression and Anxiety

Home Remedies For Losing Weight

Home Remedies For Blood Pressure and Diabetes

Home Remedies For Headaches and Insomnia

Home Remedies For Sinusitis and Tonsillitis

Home Remedies For Constipation and Diarrhea

Home Remedies For Asthma and Bronchitis

Home Remedies For Dehydration and Vomiting

Home Remedies For Pneumonia and Tuberculosis

NOTES

NOTES

NOTES

NOTES

www.ingramcontent.com/pod-product-compliance
Lightning Source LLC
Chambersburg PA
CBHW061942280526
45787CB00004B/1689